CURRY

Asian Health Food

Food

13 of the healthiest food ingredients in your favourite Eastern Food

By

John Farrell

ABOUT THE AUTHOR

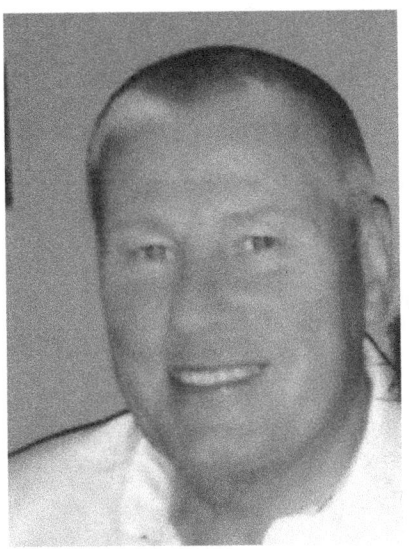

John Farrell is a qualified Mechanical Engineer. His working career has been long and varied and his skills include electrical installation, plumbing and plant maintenance at various engineering and food production plants. John has also lectured in oxy-acetylene and maual arc welding at a Manchester college. He holds licences to drive buses and coaches and in recent years has been a Senior Inspector at a Greater Manchester Bus Company and a District Manager in the local government public transport sector.

John is an authority on Chinese Martial arts and Chi Kung and still teaches these skills in Manchester England. His martial art career has spanned almost 45 years and is showing no signs of ending at this time.

Recently retired, he has also co-authored "Understanding Chi

Kung" with his brother Peter, which is available on Amazon as a paperback and also as a Kindle e- book.

ACKNOWLEDGMENTS

Thank you to my Wife, Brenda for allowing me to spend endless hours at the computer, both because of my writing and also research either through the internet or through various reference books which I continuously buy. I would also like to thank the people who provided the information whether verbal or written and even through media such as Facebook and Twitter as well as video presentations including YouTube and specific websites etc. My esteemed admiration goes to you for putting such valuable information in mediums available to the general public.

DISCLAIMER

The information presented to the readers of this book is accurate within the author's understanding of the topics of Food, Nutrition and Health. In a broad sense it is based on scientific and traditional theories and the author has attempted to find a meeting point between the two (without attempting to create a false synthesis) by drawing upon the teachings, opinions and expositions of various nutritionists and other eminent persons in associated fields. The author makes no attempt to claim that the work in the compilation is all his own and some information currently in the public domain has been used for reference. The book has been written for the information of those who are curious about the beneficial effects of the ingredients used in making curries of all kinds and from many geographical areas. It may also serve to provide a basic understanding of both ancient and modern scientific theories underlying the use of such ingredients. To this end, the reader will gain some insight into not only the use of these ingredients for flavour but also for their wider medicinal or health properties with due regard to both scientific and traditional paradigms. It is not intended as medical advice and should not be perceived as a substitute for treatment by a qualified medical practitioner. In the same vein, there is no intention to provide advice of any kind as the author simply wishes to provide an understanding of the **current** theories surrounding some remarkable curry ingredients that have, to some extent, aided his own health.

HEALTH WARNING

If you intend to embark on any nutrition program or drastic change of diet you are advised to consult a medical practitioner, particularly if you have any underlying medical conditions.

The theories presented in the text are the result of much research from sources generally thought to be experts in the field of nutrition and medical science. Some theories however may not have been subjected to the same degree of research trials and scrutiny as others but it is known that they have been major factors in folk medicine from universal sources. I only wish to elucidate the basic principles and reported effectiveness of eating these food ingredients and only encourage the use of these foods and spices etc. as a preventive and adjunctive therapy to a healthy lifestyle.

Always remember that more of something is not necessarily better and the reader is advised to research any possible contra-indications and the recommended daily amounts needed to promote and sustain a healthy life.

FOREWORD

Since my teens (many years ago) I have been a lover of Curry and having gained a taste for it I tried various flavours and types and have never really found one that I didn't like. I do have more of a regard for the ones with a good number of chilies added. I find the flavour of chilies quite addictive and have some type of hot pepper sauce with practically every other type of meal, even a roast dinner!

When I began to experiment with making my own curries at home, I made a comprehensive study of different recipes from around the world, most notably different regions of India and Pakistan. I found also that curry as a dish was also part of the diet in places like Afghanistan, some middle-eastern countries and China, Japan, Indonesia and Thailand. In fact, it is common in some form, in various parts of Asia. Each region seemed to have its own blend of spices and other ingredients. On further investigation I noted that some of the spices and ingredients used locally were indigenous to those certain areas but this did not account for the similarity of main spices used in such geographically distant places.

I spend much of my time in the Chinese community in Manchester, England, teaching Chinese Martial Arts, some of which involves understanding Chinese History and Culture. I knew that the "Silk Road" was a trade route that linked Asia with many far off places for the main purpose of trading Chinese silk however it soon became a route for the trading of all conceivable types of goods including spices from Africa, Europe, Persia and Arabia, India, China and Indonesia. It also became a route for cultural and religious exchange. With cultural exchange over a huge area it is inevitable that some facets of a particular culture, religion and technical knowledge for example will be learned and sometimes adopted by other cultures.

Botanical plant species were also traded for use in other regions along the Silk routes and these became useful as foods or food ingredients. They were also used in the preparation of medicines, ointments and as a general adjunct to health. It is interesting to note that many ancient cultures used plants, herbs and spices and other natural elements to heal and more importantly to prevent illness. It therefore seemed patently obvious to me that they would naturally use these medicinal foods etc. as an adjunct to a healthy diet.

Looking back on my own childhood I remember the use of Rose Hips as a source of vitamin C and on further reflection I saw the use of digestive aids such as Arrowroot and Ginger being used in biscuits. Dandelion and Burdock a soft drink now was originally brewed as a type of alcohol but the roots were also used to treat skin ailments and purify the blood.

These reflections prompted me to look back to Curry and see if any of those ingredients had any relationship to illness prevention and cure or as medicinal aids including to the mega-important digestive system.

During my research I have had access to various contributors, from who's experience and willingness to share with the world, I have gleaned much information and the opportunity to cross reference past and present theories and research. I am forever indebted to these people for the opportunity to understand my own health issues and compile this small book on the health benefits of some Curry ingredients. I personally have not come across a book written on this topic however I will stand corrected and humbled if one comes to light.

My extensive research has established that the body can cure itself, given the correct nutrition and the right mental attitude. It has also established that processed food and un-needed additions of colouring, flavouring and preservatives and Genetically Modified Food etc. is messing up our immune systems and thus creating bad health across the whole of the universe. We were admonished in the past to; LET FOOD BE THY MEDICINE!

Unfortunately, food manufacturers feel the need to mass produce food and add colouring to make it look more appealing and then add chemicals to ensure a longer shelf life and stop things turning rancid.

Further to this unholy equation, it seems obvious to me that Pharmaceutical companies have little or no interest in you being healthy as this would affect their monstrous profits.

AVOID PROCESSED FOOD AT ALL COSTS!!!!

Try as much as possible to eat organic produce as affordable but if it is not possible you can reduce toxicity of pesticides by peeling thick skinned produce to at least remove some of the harmful chemical on the outside. I try to clean the outside of produce with a nail type brush and wipe dry with kitchen roll to at least help remove chemical residue however I am acutely aware that such chemicals do permeate the entire product during growth.

HOW TO USE THIS BOOK

I have tried to simplify the use of this book for the reader. The book has been constructed with the use of separate chapters for each of the curry ingredients which I class as some preferred ingredients in the curries I personally like to make and eat. Within each chapter is a description of the ingredient and its genus or plant origin. Each chapter further contains a list of the chemicals derived from each ingredient and their known or supposed health benefits. Some of these benefits listed are known to have substantial research by scientists and others possibly less research but good known results so far. Others may still be the subject of ongoing research or long term studies. Many of these ingredients (and their chemicals) are known to be of practical use in Ayurvedic and Chinese traditional medicine as well as being cited as important in the traditional medicines of many other cultures.

In an effort to make it easier for the discerning reader and avoid the necessity of thumbing back through other pages, I have repeated information regarding each chemical where it also occurs within the make-up of another ingredient in each particular chapter.

Table of Contents

CHAPTER1-COMMON INGREDIENTS

MY MOST COMMON CURRY INGREDIENTS

Regionally and globally the most common curry ingredients may vary according to availability and obviously different tastes. Some do however to a greater or lesser degree seem to appear more frequently in the west and certainly in my opinion in Great Britain at least. I am using my own experience as a yardstick but I wholeheartedly expect that people who are better cooks and perhaps more informed than me, may have differing opinions. My intention is purely to bring to the attention of the uninformed or those who will not even try what they perceive as "foreign" food, that even the use of one or some of the ingredients, may enhance their diet and their health simultaneously.

To this end I put forward a list of ingredients which I use myself in my culinary efforts. I do not claim to use all the ingredients in the different curries I make and by the same rule I do not claim to make curries with the same prowess as a "Curry Chef" for example. I am confident however that all my family leave empty plates at the end of a meal!

My main ingredient list contains,
> Garlic,
> Ginger,
> Chillies,
> Fenugreek,
> Cinnamon (or Cassia Bark),
> Cardamom,

Turmeric,
Cumin,
Fennel Seeds,
Onion,
Tomatoes,
Coriander (Cilantro),
Black Peppercorn.

(There are other ingredients which I sometimes use but these will not be discussed in this volume).

In successive sections of the book I will put forward theories regarding each of the aforementioned ingredients and their perceived connection to health, based on my investigation and that of many others. Here, I again point out that concrete evidence of efficacy is difficult because extensive and conclusive research is not always readily available.

That said, I remain convinced that ABSENCE OF EVIDENCE IS NOT EVIDENCE OF ABSENCE.

CHAPTER 2-GARLIC

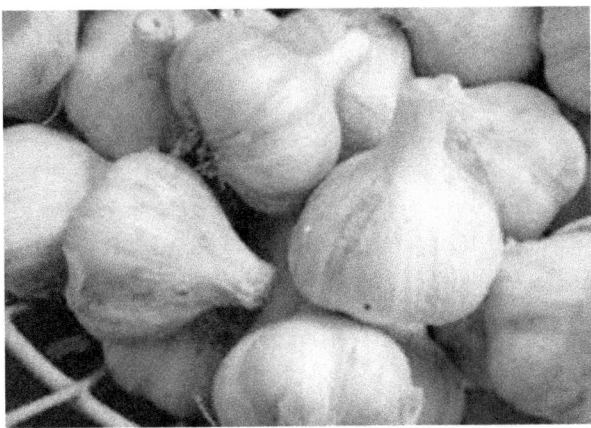

GARLIC (Allium Sativum)

Garlic is a plant from the **Allium** species and therefore is closely related to the onion and other onion tasting plants such as chives, garlic chives, leeks and shallots. It has a pungent odour and a strong taste but a wonderful flavour. It is reputed to be a curative and a preventive for many illnesses, mainly because of its chemical constituents and the individual or combined effects of these chemicals. These are;

Quercetin
(Chemical Formula C15H10O7)

Is a powerful antioxidant (available in many foods) and combats free radicals in the body. It is thought to be a powerful anti-inflammatory agent and may help to eradicate many problems associated with inflammation such as joint swelling, skin inflammation and various allergic reactions.

Vitamin C (Ascorbic Acid)
(Chemical-Formula - C6H8O6)

is a potent antioxidant and is easily soluble in the body. It is not capable of being stored in the body and so daily intake is necessary. It is necessary for cellular health, the production of collagen, the absorption of iron and promotes cell healing. Absence of vitamin C results in the poor healing of cuts and wounds and could predominantly lead to Scurvy. In the distant past Scurvy was quite common and resulted in debilitating conditions and loss of life. In modern times it is thought that lack of antioxidants such as Vitamin C could cause oxidation or oxidative damage to cells which in turn is thought to be a factor in the formation of cancer cells.

Vitamin-B(Pyroxidine)
(Chemical-Formula - C8H11NO3)

is again not able to be stored by the body but is readily available in many foods. Its function is to allow the body to convert proteins and carbohydrates into a storable energy source. Erythrocytes or red blood cells carry oxygen around the body with the aid of an integral protein called Haemoglobin which makes the process of carrying oxygen to the cells via the lungs and conversely the expiration of Carbon Dioxide via the lungs (breathing)efficient. The manufacture of Haemoglobin is initially made possible by the presence of Pyridoxine.

Manganese
(Chemical-Formula - MnO2)

is a mineral naturally occurring in our bodies in very small amounts, however it is generally agreed that this amount needs to be annexed by our dietary intake. Manganese acts as a partner agent in the production of my complicated enzymes such as manganese super oxide dismutase enzyme which is another antioxidant responsible for stopping cellular damage by free radicals. It is also involved in the production of Collagen, an essential protein for healthy skin, the musculoskeletal system and the exterior protection of some organs.

Selenium
(Chemical-Formula - Se)

Medical sources cite the mineral, Selenium as an essential mineral for bodily health and it is fortunately found in Garlic amongst many other food sources. Its selenoproteins and co-enzymes may be responsible for combatting many diseases and its depletion in the body affects the immune system and may produce a health status which allows the production of some cancers.

Allicin
(Chemical-Formula - C6H10OS2)

Is essentially an integral mechanism within garlic for its self-protection. When invaded by microbes or bacteria, Garlic produces an antimicrobial, antibacterial chemical called Allicin. This chemical has the same use in human health and is a powerful antioxidant. Research also shows that it could prevent or aid recovery from cancer as well as help to control blood pressure. It has also been found to be efficacious in the topical treatment of insect stings and bites as well as small animal bites. (May require prolonged application) Research indicates that it may also help with the treatment of cardiovascular disease and also in combatting the "common cold".

NB; Calcium, Iron, Phosphorus, Copper, Potassium and vitamin B1 are also present in lower amounts however they are equally important to the synergy involved in aiding health.

Calcium
(Chemical-Formula - Ca)

is available from many foods but processed food consumption may lessen our chances of providing the body with the amount of this essential chemical it needs to promote healthy bones and teeth. Calcium is needed for healthy growth and also to combat age related weaknesses such as Osteoporosis. Some research indicates that it may have a role in combating or preventing some types of cancer.

Iron
(Chemical-Formula - Fe)

is an integral part of red blood cells, responsible for carrying oxygen to various parts of the body. Iron helps the metabolism of proteins. A deficiency of iron will necessarily result in Anaemia because it lessens the production of red blood cells. For these same reasons it will obviously affect the proper function of every organ and cell in the body which rely on oxygen rich red blood cells for nourishment.

Phosphorus
(Chemical-Formula - P)

helps us to get the most benefit from our food in terms energy and goodness. It plays a major role in the elimination of waste from the body after it has taken the goodness from the food consumed. As with Calcium, it is a major factor in the health of bone and teeth and of major importance to the performance various organs and brain functions.

Copper
(Chemical-Formula - Cu)

is not produced by the body but is essential to include in our diet. In past times people used to use copper vessels to drink or cook because they knew it was needed in their diet. The practice of wearing copper on the body was common as it was believed to reduce the symptoms of Arthritis etc. Its synergy with other chemicals in the body does in fact result in reducing the symptomatic swelling and pain of Arthritis. It works in conjunction with iron to help produce a greater amount of red blood cells, thus helping to prevent Anaemia and the resultant lack of energy and zest for life. Copper has an effect on the health of many organs and tissues and seems to be a factor in preventing age related symptoms.

Potassium
(Chemical-Formula - K)

has a major effect on the health of the Brain and nerve function and helps to prevent stress related problems.It is well known that stress can manifest itself by affecting the nervous system and blood flow to the brain and other vital organs. It is a major factor in Hypertension (High blood Pressure) which seems to be more common in this fast-paced world we live in. An adequate supply of Potassium may stop the onset of Apoplexy (Stroke) and improving general health and vitality. A general lack of Potassium which is Electrolytic (electrically conductive) will deplete the health of the blood and major organs, leading to a reduction in muscular health and function. It also has an effect on the repair of tissues within the body.

Vitamin-B1(Thiamine)
(Chemical-Formula - $C_{12}H_{17}N_4OS$)

is known to be a factor in retarding stress related problems. It is essential to the health of the nervous system. It is instrumental in the processes of producing Glucose from Carbohydrates and processing of proteins and fats. It is known as an anti-pellagra vitamin. Pellagra, although once common was mainly associated with poorer sections of society and manifested itself with symptoms such as diarrhoea, skin rashes and general maladies including tiredness and sometimes resulted in death itself. Suffice it to say that it is essential to health and its presence in the diet has a positive effect on skin and tissue and the efficient operation of the body's waste elimination system.

CHAPTER 3-GINGER

GINGER (*Zingiber officinale*)

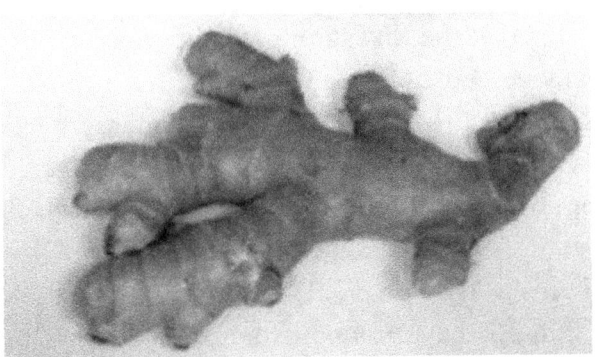

Ginger (known to the Chinese as the Man Shaped Root) is from the **Zingiberaceae** species, is low in calories and is well known in herbal and natural medicine for having anti sickness properties and alleviates suffering in travel sickness and also morning sickness in expectant mothers. It is natural and causes no known side effects to the mother or the unborn child in the way that some proprietary drugs might. It is also noted for its properties as a digestive aid. It is known to relieve pressure caused by wind (stomach or intestinal gas) and prevents intestinal cramp. It is a good source of dietary fibre and contains many vitamins and minerals (Ginger biscuits were originally made as a digestive aid). Besides having the above effects, Ginger contains chemicals known as *Gingerols* which are anti-oxidant and anti-inflammatory. Antioxidants inhibit the progress and formation of scavenging free radicals and prevent them from damaging cells and the possible formation of Cancer cells.

Ginger's anti-inflammatory effects are well tested in both herbal and western medicine whether taken internally in one's diet or used topically to alleviate symptoms like joint pain. It has the remarkable effect, when ingested of warming the whole body including the extremities and is a potent reducer of joint swelling and pain.

Some research indicates that the digestion of ginger may have a positive effect on damage caused by radiation from X rays etc. but I believe there is much more research to be done in this area.

It is thought that it can help to alleviate the symptoms of cold and flu by promoting sweating. Seemingly the advice our peers gave us about sweating Flu out may not have been that misguided as sweat helps to fight external infection!

The most notable thing I have found from researching the medicinal properties of Ginger is that laboratory tests done in the United States of America have shown a direct co-relation between Ginger (and specifically (6) Gingerol) **(Chemical Formula - $C_{17}H_{26}O_4$)** and the prevention and eradication of certain cancers researched in the trials.

My investigations seem to confirm that Ginger has no known side effects.

NB; Ground ginger is also used as a topical preparation in Chinese Medicine to alleviate joint pain and stiffness and to reduce inflammation and muscle soreness.

CHAPTER 4-CHILLIES

CHILLI PEPPERS (Capsicum)

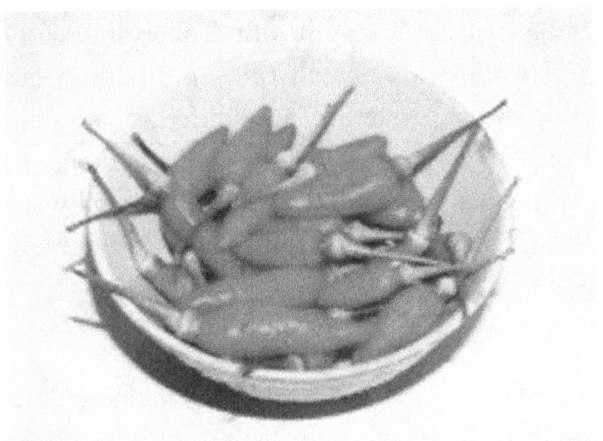

Chilli peppers of all the fruits originating from the **Capsicum** genus are the most intensely flavoured and all have different heat or intensity. This heat is measured on a scale called the Scoville scale. The heat produced by chillies can range from being pleasantly warm and flavourful to fiery and mouth numbing. In terms of medicinal properties, it is thought that the hotter the pepper, the better its efficacy, however some palates may find extremely hot peppers unbearable and even nasty. As mentioned in the Foreword to this book, I have decided is that Chillies are remarkably addictive to me personally and I like to include them in some form (including hot chilli sauce or Chilli oil) with many of my meals. Capsaicin (8-methyl-6-(E)-noneamide) is responsible for intense heat of chillies in conjunction with other chemicals in various concentrations (Dihydrocapsaicin Nordihydrocapsaicin, Homocapsaicin, Homodihydrocapsaicin). Together they are referred to as Capsaicinoids . The heat produced by these chemicals causes the mucous membranes to release fluid thus reducing sinus and nasal blockage. Another effect is the production of sweat which both cools externally and has an antibacterial effect on the surface of the skin, thus cleansing and promoting skin and body health. Taken internally in any form it is anti-parasitic and thus may aid the health of gut flora and boost the immune system. In addition, Capsaicin appears to assist the effectiveness of other natural treatments in combatting various illnesses. A study at the University of Pittsburg deduced that Capsaicin caused Apoptosis (effectively suicide) in Cancer cells studied.

Red chillies are the ripest form of chillies as they change colour during the ripening process. They are extremely high in vitamin C and B vitamins and also have lower levels of Vitamin A.($C_{20}H_{30}O$)
Added to these, they contain high levels of Iron and Potassium as well as Magnesium which is essential for the regulation of blood pressure, warding off heart and stroke problems as well as helping to prevent Osteoporosis. Studies have shown that a sufficient supply of Magnesium can influence blood sugar levels and thereby help to control the onset of Type 2 Diabetes.

Vitamin-C(AscorbicAcid)
(Chemical-Formula - $C_6H_8O_6$)

is a potent antioxidant and is easily soluble in the body. It is not capable of being stored in the body and so daily intake is necessary. It is necessary for cellular health, the production of Collagen, the absorption of iron and promotes cell healing. Absence of vitamin C results in the poor healing of cuts and wounds and could predominantly lead to Scurvy. In the distant past Scurvy was quite common and resulted in debilitating conditions and loss of life. In modern times it is thought that lack of antioxidants such as Vitamin C could cause Oxidation or oxidative damage to cells which in turn is thought to be a factor in the formation of cancer cells.

Vitamin-A
(Chemical-Formula - C20H30O)

Vitamin A is a group of nutritional compounds that includes several A provitamins and carotenoids. Vitamin A has multiple functions: it is important for human growth and for maintaining a healthy immune system and eyesight. Vitamin A has a metabolite known as Retinoic Acid which acts as a growth factor for epithelial cells which line the cavities and exterior of blood cells.

B-Vitamin Complex

Vitamin B complex, are a group of several **vitamins** that traditionally have been banded together because they have mildly similar properties and because of their distribution in natural sources, and their physiological functions, which overlap considerably. Due to its solubility in water, this group of B vitamins is similar to **vitamin C**, whereas vitamins A, D, E, and K are soluble in fat.

Most of the B vitamins are understood to be coenzymes and could be described as catalysts and therefore essential in the metabolic processes of all forms of animal life. The group of vitamins includes Vitamin B1, B2, B6 and B12 as well as others.

Iron
(Chemical-Formula - Fe)

is an integral part of red blood cells, responsible for carrying oxygen to various parts of the body. Iron helps the metabolism of proteins. A deficiency of iron will necessarily result in anaemia because it lessens the production of red blood cells. For these same reasons it will obviously affect the proper function of every organ and cell in the body which rely on oxygen rich red blood cells for nourishment.

Potassium
(Chemical-Formula - K)

has a major effect on the health of the Brain and nerve function and helps to prevent stress related problems. It is well known that stress can manifest itself by affecting the nervous system and blood flow to the brain and other vital organs. It is a major factor in Hypertension (High blood Pressure) which seems to be more common in this fast-paced world we live in. An adequate supply of Potassium may stop the onset of Apoplexy (Stroke) and improving general health and vitality. A general lack of Potassium which is Electrolytic (electrically conductive) will deplete the health of the blood and major organs, leading to a reduction in muscular health and function. It also has an effect on the repair of tissues within the body.

OTHER USES
Capsaicin is an active ingredient in many proprietary and herbal topical medicines and anti-inflammatories and provides penetrating heat and healing properties to the affected area.

CHAPTER 5-FENUGREEK

FENUGREEK SEEDS (*Trigonella foenum-graecum*)

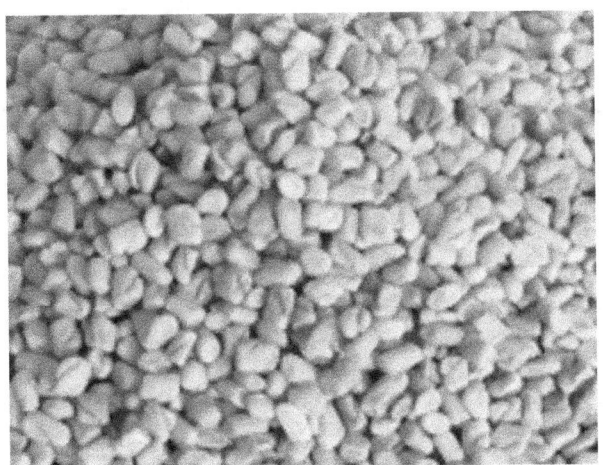

Fenugreek is a member of the **Fabaceae** genus and can be used as a herb when the leaves are dried and crushed or used fresh as an addition to casseroles or stews or even as a garnish. It is also a spice which is produced by crushing or grinding the seeds. In my opinion they could be used as a curry ingredient in any form according to taste however I think that the spice is the most convenient and most commonly used in curries. Fenugreek contains;

Iron
(Chemical-Formula - Fe)

is an integral part of red blood cells, responsible for carrying oxygen to various parts of the body. Iron helps the metabolism of proteins. A deficiency of iron will necessarily result in anaemia because it lessens the production of red blood cells. For these same reasons, it will obviously affect the proper function of every organ and cell in the body which rely on oxygen rich red blood cells for nourishment.

Magnesium
(Chemical-Formula - Mg)

Magnesium, as far as I can ascertain is one of the most important chemicals both produced and used by the body and available in many food items. It plays a huge part in the processes and health of every organ. It reacts with many other chemicals in the body and is necessary for the health of the nervous system, bone and muscle development and function and keeps the heart beating synchronously. Magnesium has the effect of regulating or balancing other chemicals in the body to ensure the correct levels for healthy organs and bodily functions including Liver and Heart Pancreas etc.

Vitamin-B6(Pyridoxine)
(Chemical-Formula - $C_8H_{11}NO_3$)

is again not able to be stored by the body but is readily available in many foods. Its function is to allow the body to convert proteins and carbohydrates into a storable energy source. Erythrocytes or red blood cells carry oxygen around the body with the aid of an integral protein called Haemoglobin which makes the process of carrying oxygen to the cells via the lungs and conversely the expiration of Carbon Dioxide via the lungs (breathing)efficient. The manufacture of Haemoglobin is initially made possible by the presence of Pyridoxine.

Potassium
(Chemical-Formula - K)

has a major effect on the health of the Brain and nerve function and helps to prevent stress related problems. It is well known that stress can manifest itself by affecting the nervous system and blood flow to the brain and other vital organs. It is a major factor in Hypertension (High blood Pressure) which seems to be more common in this fast paced world we live in. An adequate supply of Potassium may stop the onset of Apoplexy (Stroke) and improving general health and vitality. A general lack of Potassium which is Electrolytic (electrically conductive) will deplete the health of the blood and major organs, leading to a reduction in muscular health and function. It also has an effect on the repair of tissues within the body.

Calcium
(Chemical-Formula - Ca)

is available from many foods but processed food consumption may lessen our chances of providing the body with the amount of this essential chemical it needs to promote healthy bones and teeth. Calcium is needed for healthy growth and also to combat age related weaknesses such as Osteoporosis. Some research indicates that it may have a role in combating or preventing some types of cancer.

Vitamin-C(AscorbicAcid)
(Chemical-Formula - $C_6H_8O_6$)

is a potent antioxidant and is easily soluble in the body. It is not capable of being stored in the body and so daily intake is necessary. It is necessary for cellular health, the production of Collagen, the absorption of iron and promotes cell healing.

Absence of vitamin C results in the poor healing of cuts and wounds and could predominantly lead to Scurvy. In the distant past Scurvy was quite common and resulted in debilitating conditions and loss of life. In modern times it is thought that lack of antioxidants such as Vitamin C could cause Oxidation or oxidative damage to cells which in turn is thought to be a factor in the formation of cancer cells.

Sodium
(Chemical-Formula - Na)

Although Sodium is present in Common salt which many people use to a greater or lesser degree, it is necessary for the muscular and nervous system and the control of body fluids. Too much can cause hypertension or high blood pressure and too little may cause an imbalance in the body. The amount of Sodium required is relative to the needs of each individual but I personally do not use salt in cooking or add it to food as I rely on my food to provide my needs. That said, "one size does not fit all!"

Vitamin-A
(Chemical-Formula - C20H30O)

Vitamin A is not a single compound as might be deduced from the chemical formula but is made up of a group of organic compounds. Essential for the health of the immune system it is also essential for the maintenance and health of the eyes and the production of cells which line the cavities and surfaces of blood vessels and organs throughout the body. These are known as epithelial tissues.

Although there is not a great deal of verified research into the medicinal effects of this plant, there is evidence that it has been used and is used today for a variety of ailments and as an adjunct to other forms of medicine. It is known to be rich in Antioxidants which rid the body of free radicals known to cause damage to healthy cells.

From my understanding it seems to have an effect on the digestive system and helps to alleviate the reflux of stomach acids. As most of the immune system is located in the gut, it is totally feasible that if it helps with the digestive system then the healthy immune system can eradicate many health problems and promote amongst other things, a healthy metabolism.

Although this may be anecdotal, it is claimed that Fenugreek is used to increase male sexual desire and prowess. In females it has long been used to promote the flow of mother's milk during breastfeeding. Of extreme importance, it is also thought to be an aid to the prevention of certain types of cancer and helps to lower blood sugar by lowering the rate of absorption of sugars in the body. This is also of particular importance to those who may suffer from Diabetes. It is worth noting that is often added to proprietary medicines used to help alleviate the symptoms of coughs and Bronchitis. There are also accounts of it being used as an aid to problems caused by some vitamin deficiencies.

CHAPTER 6-CINNAMON

CINNAMON or CASSIA BARK

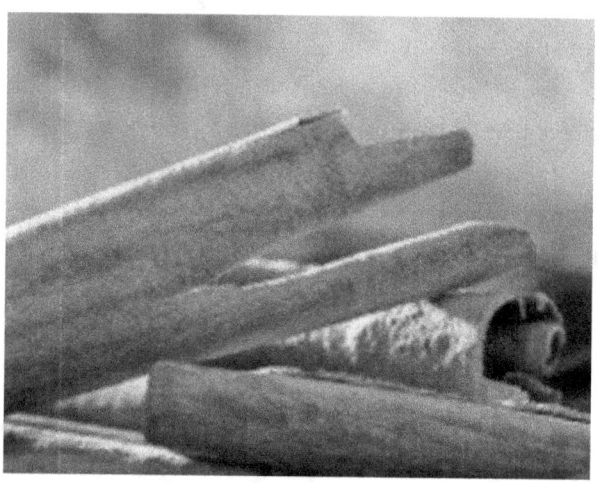

Both from the **Cinnamomum** genus, Cinnamon and Cassia bark are different but Cassia Bark is often wrongly sold as Cinnamon. Although similar, Cassia bark has a higher level of a Phytochemical called Coumarin.

Coumarin
(Chemical-Formula - C9H6O2).

Coumarin is found in many other plants but high levels or sustained use of high levels can have a detrimental effect on the liver. (This substance also has limited use in some medical treatments such as Asthma and Lymphedema according to one source) **WARNING**; In some people, even small amounts of Coumarin can have a bad effect on the liver however this seems to be a small minority of people and the effect can be reversed with treatment.

In general food use Cinnamon and Cassia are both thought to be beneficial in the control of blood sugar in the case of Diabetes. Control of blood sugar does not put the body into fat storing mode and subsequently may be instrumental in weight loss. More importantly it is evident that cancers feed on sugar and controlling blood sugar helps to stop cancers growing. (Good advice is to control your intake of refined sugars which are particularly evident in processed foods of any kind).

Much research has been done on these subjects but medical advice should still be followed in all cases and a good nutrition plan should be observed.

There is a huge amount of evidential support for the role of Cinnamon in not only the prevention of Cancers but also in fighting infection. It is a very effective Anti-oxidant and thus reduces the likelihood of the formation of cancer cells and any other cells which try to attack the body and its functions. It is widely known that that some yeast and fungal infections can be controlled by Cinnamon preparations when proprietary medicines fail. A solution of Cinnamon and hot water makes a powerful disinfectant agent which has the ability to destroy even bacteria such as E.Coli although Cinnamon bark oil is much stronger and more effective. Taken internally in food there is nothing works better to control stomach bugs caused by bacteria such as Salmonella and the eradication of such bacteria can promote health in the Gastro Intestinal Tract. The effect of this better heath can be to alleviate stomach cramps, irritable bowel syndrome and excess gas.

Cinnamon is also another Curry ingredient which contains a good amount of Manganese and thus acts with other chemicals to help to maintain the health of the body.

Manganese
(Chemical-Formula - MnO2)

is a mineral naturally occurring in our bodies in very small amounts, however it is generally agreed that this amount needs to be annexed by our dietary intake. Manganese acts as a partner agent in the production of my complicated enzymes such as manganese super oxide dismutase enzyme which is another antioxidant responsible for stopping cellular damage by free radicals. It is also involved in the production of Collagen, an essential protein for healthy skin, the musculoskeletal system and the exterior protection of some organs.

CHAPTER 7 -CARDAMOM

GREEN CARDAMOM (<u>Elettaria cardamomum</u>)

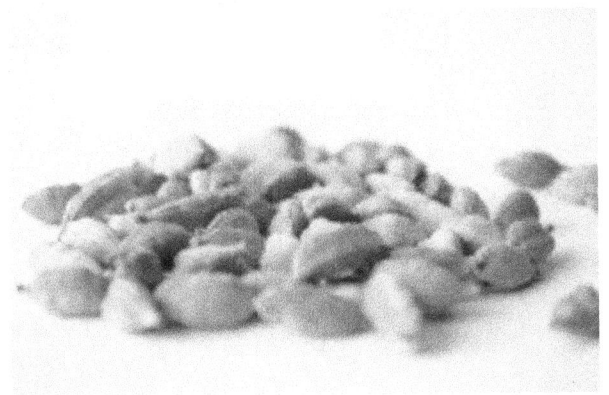

Green Cardamom from the genus **Zingiberaceae** is a part of the Ginger family and is widely used throughout the far east for not only its cooking and taste properties but is also regarded as a potent medicine. It is chewed as a breath freshener and is commonly used in proprietary Breath Fresheners and some toothpastes. The reasons for this are twofold as cardamom is known to be beneficial in the treatment of mouth ulcers and gum infections as well as being regarded as a potent preventative for respiratory problems. In China it can be an ingredient in many herbal medicines and is widely thought to be effective in reducing Gastro-intestinal disorders as is its relative, Ginger.

The essential oils found in Cardamom very dependent on where they are grown however it is widely thought that these oils such as a-terpinol, myrcene and limonine have antioxidant properties which prevent damage to cells. In the same vein tests are revealing that it may be effective in the treatment and cure of certain types of cancers and the apoptosis or programmed (cancer) cell death however more research needs to be done before definite claims as to its efficacy can be made. It is however known to be anti-inflammatory and anti-fungal. Chinese and Indian medical herbalists seem to agree that it is useful in the control of blood pressure by it fibrous action of cleaning inside blood vessels and arteries.

CHAPTER 8-TURMERIC

TURMERIC ROOT AND POWDER (Curcuma Longa)

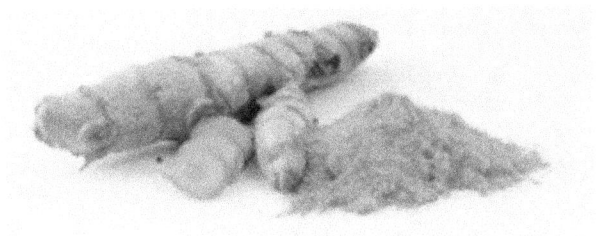

An Indian wonder ingredient! This humble root from the genus **Curcuma,** has long been regarded as a panacea. Its health benefits have become known worldwide for the cure and prevention of many ailments. Studies show that it contains compounds known as Curcuminoids. The most notable of these is Curcumin which is another potent antioxidant helping to control the damaging power of free radicals. It also aids the body's power to produce its own antioxidants, again helping to control the cellular damage caused by free radicals.

Curcumin
(Chemical-Formula - $C_{21}H_{20}O_6$)
has the quality of being anti-inflammatory particularly in the case of chronic inflammation.Chronic inflammation, according to scientific studies is a major factor in the cause if many debilitating diseases and conditions. Its effects appear to stop the onset of degenerative diseases such as Alzheimer's, degenerative heart disease and Cancer by its action at a molecular level. The anti-inflammatory properties of Curcumin compare favourably with those of proprietary drugs and have no apparent side effects.

Curcumin is relatively low in volume in Turmeric so it requires the boosting catalyst, Piperine to make it more effective. **(See Black Peppercorns)**

CHAPTER 9-CUMIN

CUMIN SEEDS (Cuminum cyminum)

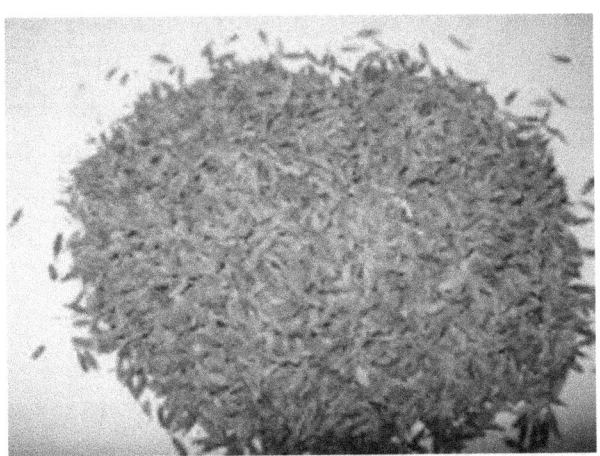

Cumin is from the genus **Umbelliferae**. Besides being an ingredient in Curry Powder, Cumin is widely used in Mexican, Middle Eastern and North African cookery. It has a sort of pepper like taste but a much more pungent flavour. It is a very noticeable flavour in curry and has a rich aroma when cooked.it can be used whole as a seed but blends better when ground in a pestle and mortar or spice grinder.

Nutritionally it is high in **Iron,** which is a major factor in carrying oxygenated red blood cells to the various parts of the body and promoting and ensuring the health of cells and the immune system. Iron is essential to top up the energy level of the body and low levels produce extreme tiredness and lethargy. It also contains the chemicals and vitamins listed below, after **Iron;**

Iron
(Chemical-Formula - Fe)

is an integral part of red blood cells, responsible for carrying oxygen to various parts of the body. Iron helps the metabolism of proteins. A deficiency of iron will necessarily result in anaemia because it lessens the production of red blood cells. For these same reasons it will obviously affect the proper function of every organ and cell in the body which rely on oxygen rich red blood cells for nourishment.

Manganese
(Chemical-Formula - MnO2)

is a mineral naturally occurring in our bodies in very small amounts however it is generally agreed that this amount needs to be annexed by our dietary intake. Manganese acts as a partner agent in the production of my complicated enzymes such as manganese super oxide dismutase enzyme which is another antioxidant responsible for stopping cellular damage by free radicals. It is also involved in the production of Collagen, an essential protein for healthy skin, the musculoskeletal system and the exterior protection of some organs.

Copper
(Chemical-Formula - Cu)

is not produced by the body but is essential to include in our diet. In past times people used to use copper vessels to drink or cook because they knew it was needed in our diet. The practice of wearing copper on the body was common as it was believed to reduce the symptoms of Arthritis etc. Its synergy with other chemicals in the body does in fact result in reducing the symptomatic swelling and pain of Arthritis. It works in conjunction with iron to help produce a greater amount of red blood cells, thus helping to prevent Anaemia and the resultant lack of energy and zest for life. Copper has an effect on the health of many organs and tissues and seems to be a factor in preventing age related symptoms.

Calcium
(Chemical-Formula - Ca)

is available from many foods but processed food consumption may lessen our chances of providing the body with the amount of this essential chemical it needs to promote healthy bones and teeth. Calcium is needed for healthy growth and also to combat age related weaknesses such as Osteoporosis. Some research indicates that it may have a role in combating or preventing some types of cancer.

Magnesium
(Chemical-Formula - Mg)

Magnesium, as far as I can ascertain is one of the most important chemicals both produced and used by the body and available in many food items. It plays a huge part in the processes and health of every organ. It reacts with many other chemicals in the body and is necessary for the health of the nervous system, bone and muscle development and function and keeps the heart beating synchronously. Magnesium has the effect of regulating or balancing other chemicals in the body to ensure the correct levels for healthy organs and bodily functions including Liver and Heart Pancreas etc.

Vitamin-B1(Thiamine)
(Chemical-Formula - C12H17N4OS+)

is known to be a factor in retarding stress related problems. It is essential to the health of the nervous system. It is instrumental in the processes of producing Glucose from Carbohydrates and processing of proteins and fats. It is known as an anti-pellagra vitamin. Pellagra, although once common was mainly associated with poorer sections of society and manifested itself with symptoms such as diarrhoea, skin rashes and general maladies including tiredness and sometimes resulted in death itself. Suffice it to say that it is essential to health and its presence in the diet has a positive effect on skin and tissue and the efficient operation of the body's waste elimination system.

Phosphorus
(Chemical-Formula - P)

helps us to get the most benefit from our food in terms energy and goodness. It plays a major role in the elimination of waste from the body after it has the goodness from the food consumed. As with Calcium, it is a major factor in the health of bone and teeth and of major importance to the performance various organs and brain functions. Its various associations with romance, love and potency as an aphrodisiac in times gone by, belie its qualities as a potent digestive aid, liver tonic and free radical scavenger. These qualities make it another soldier in the fight against the production of cancer cells in the body.

CHAPTER 10-FENNEL SEEDS

FENNEL SEEDS (*Foeniculum vulgare*)

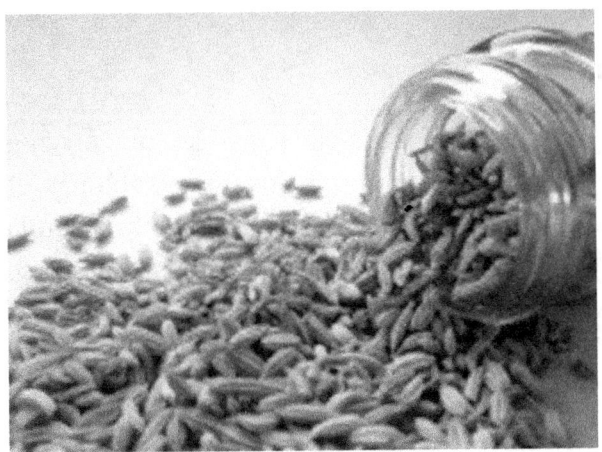

From the flowering plant, Fennel of the **Foeniculum** genus, the seeds taste a little like aniseed and are often chewed in India, Pakistan and surrounding areas of the continent to aid digestion and to freshen breath. The essential oils help to promote the secretion of digestive juices. This and the fact that it is mildly laxative and reduces inflammation in the stomach help to prevent gastro-intestinal problems such as Irritable Bowel Syndrome and Constipation and reduce the likelihood of other major or minor issues caused by blockages in the intestines. Fennel seeds have been shown to contain dietary fibre which also help with digestion and elimination.

Some of these issues may in time lead to cancerous tumors being formed and Fennel has a proven beneficial effect on minimizing or preventing their growth. Scientific tests also reveal that it is beneficial in dealing with the harmful effects caused by radiation treatment in cancer patients. Various preparations of the seed are used to prevent some breast and liver cancer. The seeds are known to contain many health promoting vitamins and antioxidants such as;

Iron
(Chemical-Formula - Fe)

is an integral part of red blood cells, responsible for carrying oxygen to various parts of the body. Iron helps the metabolism of proteins. A deficiency of iron will necessarily result in anaemia because it lessens the production of red blood cells. For these same reasons, it will obviously affect the proper function of every organ and cell in the body which rely on oxygen rich red blood cells for nourishment.

Potassium
(Chemical-Formula - K)

has a major effect on the health of the Brain and nerve function and helps to prevent stress related problems. It is well known that stress can manifest itself by affecting the nervous system and blood flow to the brain and other vital organs. It is a major factor in Hypertension (High blood Pressure) which seems to be more common in this fast paced world we live in. An adequate supply of Potassium may stop the onset of Apoplexy (Stroke) and improving general health and vitality. A general lack of Potassium which is Electrolytic (electrically conductive) will deplete the health of the blood and major organs, leading to a reduction in muscular health and function. It also has an effect on the repair of tissues within the body.

Copper
(Chemical-Formula - Cu)

Copper is not produced by the body but is essential to include in our diet. In past times people used to use copper vessels to drink or cook because they knew it was needed in our diet. The practice of wearing copper on the body was common as it was believed to reduce the symptoms of Arthritis etc. Its synergy with other chemicals in the body does in fact result in reducing the symptomatic swelling and pain of Arthritis. It works in conjunction with iron to help produce a greater amount of red blood cells, thus helping to prevent Anaemia and the resultant lack of energy and zest for life. Copper has an effect on the health of many organs and tissues and seems to be a factor in preventing age related symptoms.

Zinc
(Chemical-Formula - Zn)

Zinc is not readily stored in the body but is essential to the immune system and the development and repair of the human body. It is a factor in many cellular functions and enables wound healing and protein assimilation as well. It is also known to be beneficial in warding off seasonal colds etc. and is thought to be beneficial in repairing heart disease and benefitting Diabetes sufferers.

Selenium
(Chemical-Formula - Se)

Medical sources cite the mineral, Selenium as an essential mineral for bodily health and it is fortunately found in Garlic amongst many other food sources. Its selenoproteins and co-enzymes may be responsible for combating many diseases and its depletion in the body affects the immune system and may produce a health status which allows the production of some cancers.

Magnesium
(Chemical-Formula - Mg)

Magnesium, as far as I can ascertain is one of the most important chemicals both produced and used by the body and available in many food items. It plays a huge part in the processes and health of every organ. It reacts with many other chemicals in the body and is necessary for the health of the nervous system, bone and muscle development and function and keeps the heart beating synchronously. Magnesium has the effect of regulating or balancing other chemicals in the body to ensure the correct levels for healthy organs and bodily functions including Liver and Heart Pancreas etc.

Vitamin-C(AscorbicAcid)
(Chemical-Formula - $C_6H_8O_6$)

is a potent antioxidant and is easily soluble in the body. It is not capable of being stored in the body and so daily intake is necessary. It is necessary for cellular health, the production of Collagen, the absorption of iron and promotes cell healing. Absence of vitamin C results in the poor healing of cuts and wounds and could predominantly lead to Scurvy. In the distant past Scurvy was quite common and resulted in debilitating conditions and loss of life. In modern times, it is thought that lack of antioxidants such as Vitamin C could cause Oxidation or oxidative damage to cells which in turn is thought to be a factor in the formation of cancer cells.

Vitamin-A

(Chemical-Formula - C20H30O)

Vitamin A is a group of nutritional compounds that includes several A provitamins and carotenoids. Vitamin A has multiple functions: it is important for human growth and for maintaining a healthy immune system and eyesight. Vitamin A has a metabolite known as Retinoic Acid which acts as a growth factor for epithelial cells which line the cavities and exterior of blood cells.

Vitamin-E(AlphaTocopherol)
(Chemical-Formula - C29H50O2)

Vitamin E is available in a multitude of forms however Alpha Tocopherol is the only useful form for humans. Antioxidant in nature it is only available as an adjunct to human diet and thus helps rid the body of free radicals and protects against toxins. Vitamin E has a beneficial effect the prevention of diabetes and is thought to be helpful in the fight against the onset of such disorders as Alzheimer's Disease and other neurological problems.

CHAPTER 11-ONIONS

ONIONS (Allium cepa)

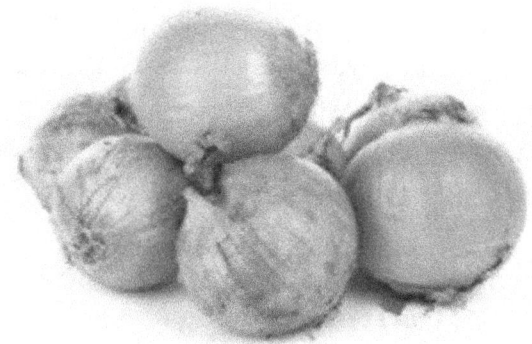

Onions are another member of the **Allium** family and are highly regarded for their heath promoting and curative properties. They have a strong odour because they contain Sulphur compounds known as Allyl Sulphides. Onions have the highest Quercetin content of all the Allium vegetables but some of this may be drastically decreased by peeling too many layers before cooking or other uses. Quercetin is known to be particularly useful in the treatment of Cancers particularly when onions are used regularly or on a daily basis. Cooking does not degrade the amount of Quercetin as it is absorbed in the cooking liquids.

Onions potentially help to eradicate bacteria in the body when taken orally and may also lessen scar tissue when applied topically. There is also much evidence that onions can have a marked effect on the health of the heart, skeletal system and the reduction of inflammation. All in all, Onions are what I regard as a Superfood.

Quercetin
(Chemical-Formula - C15H10O7)

Is a powerful antioxidant (available in many foods) and combats free radicals in the body. It is thought to be a powerful anti-inflammatory agent and may help to eradicate many problems associated with inflammation such as joint swelling, skin inflammation and various allergic reactions.

Vitamin-B7 (Biotin)
(Chemical-Formula - C10H16N2O3S)

Sometimes referred to as Vitamin H, it keeps the skin, nails and hair in good condition. It is also essential in the maintenance of the nervous system. Lack of this vitamin can result in rough and cracked skin and even depression. This however is more likely in people who have other medical problems caused by excesses of body assaulting habits such as excessive alcohol etc.

Manganese
(Chemical-Formula - MnO2)

is a mineral naturally occurring in our bodies in very small amounts however it is generally agreed that this amount needs to be annexed by our dietary intake. Manganese acts as a partner agent in the production of my complicated enzymes such as manganese super oxide dismutase enzyme which is another antioxidant responsible for stopping cellular damage by free radicals. It is also involved in the production of Collagen, an essential protein for healthy skin, the musculoskeletal system and the exterior protection of some organs.

Copper
(Chemical-Formula - Cu)

Copper is not produced by the body but is essential to include in our diet. In past times people used to use copper vessels to drink or cook because they knew it was needed in our diet. The practice of wearing copper on the body was common as it was believed to reduce the symptoms of Arthritis etc. Its synergy with other chemicals in the body does in fact result in reducing the symptomatic swelling and pain of Arthritis. It works in conjunction with iron to help produce a greater amount of red blood cells, thus helping to prevent anaemia and the resultant lack of energy and zest for life. Copper has an effect on the health of many organs and tissues and seems to be a factor in preventing age related symptoms.

Vitamin-B6 (Pyridoxine)
(Chemical-Formula - $C_8H_{11}NO_3$)
is again not able to be stored by the body but is readily available in many foods. Its function is to allow the body to convert proteins and carbohydrates into a storable energy source. Erythrocytes or red blood cells carry oxygen around the body with the aid of an integral protein called Haemoglobin which makes the process of carrying oxygen to the cells via the lungs and conversely the expiration of Carbon Dioxide via the lungs (breathing)efficient. The manufacture of Haemoglobin is initially made possible by the presence of Pyridoxine.

Vitamin-C(AscorbicAcid)
(Chemical-Formula - $C_6H_8O_6$)

is a potent antioxidant and is easily soluble in the body. It is not capable of being stored in the body and so daily intake is necessary. It is necessary for cellular health, the production of Collagen, the absorption of iron and promotes cell healing. Absence of vitamin C results in the poor healing of cuts and wounds and could predominantly lead to Scurvy. In the distant past Scurvy was quite common and resulted in debilitating conditions and loss of life. In modern times it is thought that lack of antioxidants such as Vitamin C could cause Oxidation or oxidative damage to cells which in turn is thought to be a factor in the formation of cancer cells.

Phosphorus
(Chemical-Formula - P)

helps us to get the most benefit from our food in terms energy and goodness. It plays a major role in the elimination of waste from the body after it has the goodness from the food consumed. As with Calcium, it is a major factor in the health of bone and teeth and of major importance to the performance various organs and brain functions.

Potassium
(Chemical-Formula - K)

has a major effect on the health of the Brain and nerve function and helps to prevent stress related problems. It is well known that stress can manifest itself by affecting the nervous system and blood flow to the brain and other vital organs. It is a major factor in Hypertension (High blood Pressure) which seems to be more common in this fast paced world we live in. An adequate supply of Potassium may stop the onset of Apoplexy (Stroke) and improving general health and vitality. A general lack of Potassium which is Electrolytic (electrically conductive) will deplete the health of the blood and major organs, leading to a reduction in muscular health and function. It also has an effect on the repair of tissues within the body.

Vitamin-B1(Thiamine)
(Chemical-Formula - $C_{12}H_{17}N_4OS$)

is known to be a factor in retarding stress related problems. It is essential to the health of the nervous system. It is instrumental in the processes of producing Glucose from Carbohydrates and processing of proteins and fats. It is known as an anti-pellagra vitamin. Pellagra, although once common was mainly associated with poorer sections of society and manifested itself with symptoms such as diarrhoea, skin rashes and general maladies including tiredness and sometimes resulted in death itself. Suffice it to say that it is essential to health and its presence in the diet has a positive effect on skin and tissue and the efficient operation of the body's waste elimination system.

Folate
(Chemical-Formula - $C_{19}H_{19}N_7O_6$)
Is a B complex vitamin which helps the production and upkeep of cells and maintains the healthy structure of DNA. It may be used in conjunction with other substances as a preventative and treatment for anemia.

CHAPTER 12-TOMATOES

TOMATOES

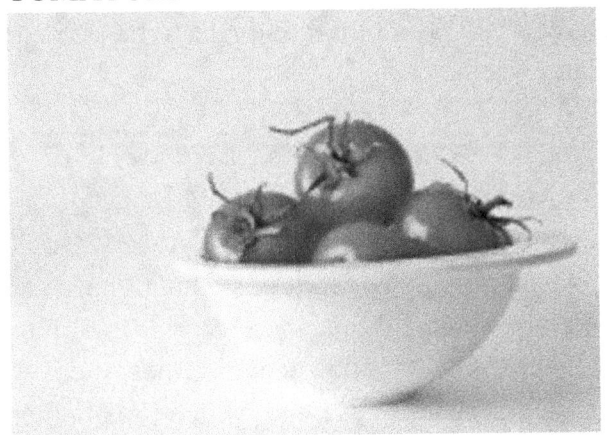

TOMATOES (*Lycopersicon esculentum.*) are from the **Solanaceae** (or Nightshade) genus and although they seem to be classed as a vegetable, the tomato is actually a fruit. In my opinion they are a "Superfruit" because they are packed with many nutrients. A rich source of antioxidants such as Lycopene and Beta-carotene, they are a veritable powerhouse in the fight against many diseases and illnesses as can be shown from the list below;

Vitamin-C (Ascorbic Acid)
(Chemical-Formula - C6H8O6)
is a potent antioxidant and is easily soluble in the body. It is not capable of being stored in the body and so daily intake is necessary. It is necessary for cellular health, the production of Collagen, the absorption of iron and promotes cell healing. Absence of vitamin C results in the poor healing of cuts and wounds and could predominantly lead to Scurvy. In the distant

past Scurvy was quite common and resulted in debilitating conditions and loss of life. n modern times it is thought that lack of antioxidants such as Vitamin C could cause Oxidation or oxidative damage to cells which in turn is thought to be a factor in the formation of cancer cells.

Manganese
(Chemical-Formula - MnO2)

is a mineral naturally occurring in our bodies in very small amounts however it is generally agreed that this amount needs to be annexed by our dietary intake. Manganese acts as a partner agent in the production of my complicated enzymes such as manganese super oxide dismutase enzyme which is another antioxidant responsible for stopping cellular damage by free radicals. It is also involved in the production of Collagen, an essential protein for healthy skin, the musculoskeletal system and the exterior protection of some organs.

Potassium
(Chemical-Formula - K)

has a major effect on the health of the Brain and nerve function and helps to prevent stress related problems. It is well known that stress can manifest itself by affecting the nervous system and blood flow to the brain and other vital organs. It is a major factor in Hypertension (High blood Pressure) which seems to be more common in this fast paced world we live in. An adequate supply of Potassium may stop the onset of Apoplexy (Stroke) and improving general health and vitality. A general lack of Potassium which is Electrolytic (electrically conductive) will deplete the health of the blood and major organs, leading to a reduction in muscular health and function. It also has an effect on the repair of tissues within the body.

Magnesium
(Chemical-Formula - Mg)

Magnesium, as far as I can ascertain is one of the most important chemicals both produced and used by the body and available in many food items. It plays a huge part in the processes and health of every organ. It reacts with many other chemicals in the body and is necessary for the health of the nervous system, bone and muscle development and function and keeps the heart beating synchronously. Magnesium has the effect of regulating or balancing other chemicals in the body to ensure the correct levels for healthy organs and bodily functions including Liver and Heart Pancreas etc.

Copper
(Chemical-Formula - Cu)

Copper is not produced by the body but is essential to include in our diet. In past times people used to use copper vessels to drink or cook because they knew it was needed in our diet. The practice of wearing copper on the body was common as it was believed to reduce the symptoms of Arthritis etc. Its synergy with other chemicals in the body does in fact result in reducing the symptomatic swelling and pain of Arthritis. It works in conjunction with iron to help produce a greater amount of red blood cells, thus helping to prevent anaemia and the resultant lack of energy and zest for life. Copper has an effect on the health of many organs and tissues and seems to be a factor in preventing age related symptoms.

Vitamin-B7 (Biotin)
(Chemical-Formula - C10H16N2O3S)

Sometimes referred to as Vitamin H, it keeps the skin, nails and hair in good condition. It is also essential in the maintenance of the nervous system. Lack of this vitamin can result in rough and cracked skin and even depression. This however is more likely in people who have other medical problems caused by excesses of body assaulting habits such as excessive alcohol etc.

Iron
(Chemical-Formula - Fe)

is an integral part of red blood cells, responsible for carrying oxygen to various parts of the body. Iron helps the metabolism of proteins. A deficiency of iron will necessarily result in anaemia because it lessens the production of red blood cells. For these same reasons it will obviously affect the proper function of every organ and cell in the body which rely on oxygen rich red blood cells for nourishment.

Zinc
(Chemical-Formula - Zn)

Zinc is not readily stored in the body but is essential to the immune system and the development and repair of the human body. It is a factor in many cellular functions and enables wound healing and protein assimilation as well. It is also known to be beneficial in warding off seasonal colds etc. and is thought to be beneficial in repairing heart disease and benefitting Diabetes sufferers.

Vitamin-A
(Chemical-Formula - C20H30O)

Vitamin A is not a single compound as might be deduced from the chemical formula but is made up of a group of organic compounds. Essential for the health of the immune system it is also essential for the maintenance and health of the eyes and the production of cells which line the cavities and surfaces of blood vessels and organs throughout the body. These are known as epithelial tissues.

Vitamin-B6(Pyridoxine)
(Chemical-Formula - C8H11NO3)

is again not able to be stored by the body but is readily available in many foods. Its function is to allow the body to convert proteins and carbohydrates into a storable energy source. Erythrocytes or red blood cells carry oxygen around the body with the aid of an integral protein called Haemoglobin which makes the process of carrying oxygen to the cells via the lungs and conversely the expiration of Carbon Dioxide via the lungs (breathing)efficient. The manufacture of Haemoglobin is initially made possible by the presence of Pyridoxine.

Folate
(Chemical-Formula - C19H19N7O6)

Is a B complex vitamin which helps the production and upkeep of cells and maintains the healthy structure of DNA. It may be used in conjunction with other substances as a preventative and treatment for anemia.

Phosphorus
(Chemical-Formula - P)
helps us to get the most benefit from our food in terms energy and goodness. It plays a major role in the elimination of waste from the body after it has the goodness from the food consumed. As with Calcium, it is a major factor in the health of bone and teeth and of major importance to the performance various organs and brain functions.

Vitamin-B1 (Thiamine)
(Chemical-Formula - C12H17N4OS+)
is known to be a factor in retarding stress related problems. It is essential to the health of the nervous system. It is instrumental in the processes of producing Glucose from Carbohydrates and processing of proteins and fats. It is known as an anti-pellagra vitamin. Pellagra, although once common was mainly associated with poorer sections of society and manifested itself with symptoms such as diarrhoea, skin rashes and general maladies including tiredness and sometimes resulted in death itself. Suffice it to say that it is essential to health and its presence in the diet has a positive effect on skin and tissue and the efficient operation of the body's waste elimination system.

Vitamin-E (Alpha Tocopherol)
(Chemical-Formula - C29H50O2)
Vitamin E is available in a multitude of forms however Alpha Tocopherol is the only useful form for humans. Antioxidant in nature it is only available as an adjunct to human diet and thus

helps rid the body of free radicals and protects against toxins. Vitamin E has a beneficial effect the prevention of diabetes and is thought to be helpful in the fight against the onset of such disorders as Alzheimer's Disease and other neurological problems.

Molybdenum
(Chemical-Formula - Mo)

Molybdenum helps in the process of waste management and elimination in the body by breaking down toxins left over from the digestive process however it main job is to assist in the breakdown of amino acids by acting as a catalyst in this biochemical process.

Vitamin-K
(Chemical-Formula - $C_{31}H_{46}O_2$)

This vitamin is actually known as vitamin K1 as there are several forms of this vitamin. Only K1 is mentioned here as it is the one which is synthesized from plants.

Vitamin K is necessary to synthesize proteins involved in blood clotting and is also essential for the synthesis of certain other proteins such as those involved in building strong bones.

Vitamin-B3 (Niacin)
(Chemical-Formula - $C_6H_5NO_2$)

Niacin is essential to the Cardiovascular system as it helps to maintain the correct level of good cholesterol. It helps to ensure the brain is healthy and is thought to a factor in the prevention of diabetes.

Chromium
(Chemical-Formula - Cr)

Chromium is only used by the body in very tiny amounts however even though this is the case it is essential in the process of metabolizing fats, carbohydrates and proteins and other biochemical processes such as the regulation of blood sugar and helps insulin perform its function.

Choline
(Chemical-Formula - C5H14NO)

Choline is a macronutrient (required in large amounts in the body) that's important to sustain the performance of a healthy metabolism and maintain good energy levels. It is essential for the health and maintenance of the liver and its processes, brain and nerve health and development and keeping the body's musculature in good health and working order.

Vitamin-B5 (Pantothenic acid)
(Chemical-Formula - C9H17NO5)

As with the rest of the B Vitamin complex, B5 helps in the metabolism of food, the health of the liver, skin, hair and eyesight. More importantly B5 is essential for the production of red blood cells, the synthesis of cholesterol in the body and the health of the digestive tract.

CHAPTER 13 CORIANDER

CORIANDER (AKA Cilantro)

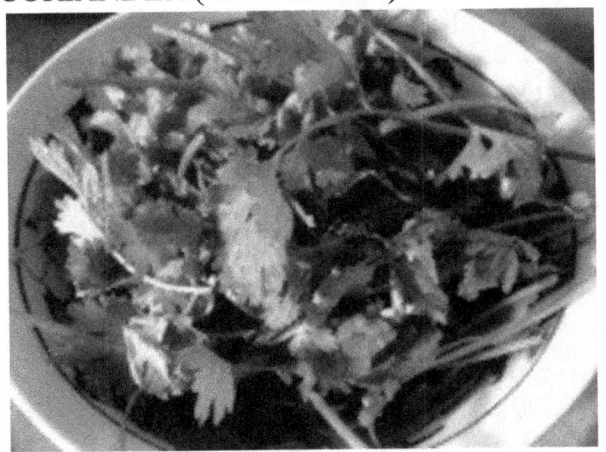

From the genus **Coriandrum** you either love it or you hate it but medicinally it is a panacea. The herb leaves and stalks can be used as a garnish in curry or the spice obtained from the seeds of the plant can be ground and added to the spice mix. The plant has quite a pungent taste and smell but it is an acquired taste.As a whole plant including the seeds it is known to have detoxification properties and helps to rid the body of heavy metals found in our food and water and even in vaccinations such as the Flu Jab, commonly given to older people. Cooking in aluminium utensils increases the levels of aluminium in the body. I dread to imagine what other toxins we are being fed in our diet, including so called "Fresh Produce"! Fortunately coriander also has anti-fungal and anti-bacterial properties and is also a digestive aid. When it is considered that a large proportion of the body's immune system is in the gut this is a huge bonus to our health. Coriander contains many antioxidants and is known to be potent in reducing the risk of cancer cell formation and also reduces the risk of inflammation. Chemically this plant has a great source of many important vitamins and minerals. Some of these are listed below;

Vitamin-A
(Chemical-Formula - $C_{20}H_{30}O$)

Vitamin A is not a single compound as might be deduced from the chemical formula but is made up of a group of organic compounds. Essential for the health of the immune system it is also essential for the maintenance and health of the eyes and the production of cells which line the cavities and surfaces of blood vessels and organs throughout the body. These are known as epithelial tissues.

Vitamin-C(AscorbicAcid)
(Chemical-Formula - $C_6H_8O_6$)

is a potent antioxidant and is easily soluble in the body. It is not capable of being stored in the body and so daily intake is necessary. It is necessary for cellular health, the production of Collagen, the absorption of iron and promotes cell healing. Absence of vitamin C results in the poor healing of cuts and wounds and could predominantly lead to Scurvy. In the distant past Scurvy was quite common and resulted in debilitating conditions and loss of life. In modern times it is thought that lack of antioxidants such as Vitamin C could cause Oxidation or oxidative damage to cells which in turn is thought to be a factor in the formation of cancer cells.

Vitamin-K
(Chemical-Formula - $C_{31}H_{46}O_2$)

This vitamin is actually known as vitamin K1 as there are several forms of this vitamin. Only K1 is mentioned here as it is the one which is synthesized from plants.

Vitamin K is necessary to synthesize proteins involved in blood clotting and is also essential for the synthesis of certain other proteins such as those involved in building strong bones.

Vitamin-E(AlphaTocopherol)
(Chemical-Formula-$C_{29}H_{50}O_2$)

Vitamin E is available in a multitude of forms however Alpha Tocopherol is the only useful form for humans. Antioxidant in nature it is only available as an adjunct to human diet and thus helps rid the body of free radicals and protects against toxins. Vitamin E has a beneficial effect the prevention of diabetes and is thought to be helpful in the fight against the onset of such disorders as Alzheimer's Disease and other neurological problems.

Manganese
(Chemical-Formula - MnO_2)

is a mineral naturally occurring in our bodies in very small amounts however it is generally agreed that this amount needs to be annexed by our dietary intake. Manganese acts as a partner agent in the production of my complicated enzymes such as manganese super oxide dismutase enzyme which is another antioxidant responsible for stopping cellular damage by free radicals. It is also involved in the production of Collagen, an essential protein for healthy skin, the musculoskeletal system and the exterior protection of some organs.

Potassium
(Chemical-Formula - K)

has a major effect on the health of the Brain and nerve function and helps to prevent stress related problems. It is well known that stress can manifest itself by affecting the nervous system and blood flow to the brain and other vital organs. It is a major factor in Hypertension (High blood Pressure) which seems to be more common in this fast-paced world we live in. An adequate supply of Potassium may stop the onset of Apoplexy (Stroke) and improving general health and vitality. A general lack of Potassium which is Electrolytic (electrically conductive) will deplete the health of the blood and major organs, leading to a reduction in muscular health and function. It also has an effect on the repair of tissues within the body.

Iron
(Chemical-Formula-Fe)

is an integral part of red blood cells, responsible for carrying oxygen to various parts of the body. Iron helps the metabolism of proteins. A deficiency of iron will necessarily result in anaemia because it lessens the production of red blood cells. For these same reasons it will obviously affect the proper function of every organ and cell in the body which rely on oxygen rich red blood cells for nourishment.

Sodium
(Chemical-FormulaNa)

Although Sodium is present in Common salt which many people use to a greater or lesser degree, it is necessary for the muscular and nervous system and the control of body fluids. Too much can cause hypertension or high blood pressure and too little may cause an imbalance in the body. The amount of Sodium required is relative to the needs of each individual but I personally do not use salt in cooking or add it to food as I rely on my food to provide my needs. That said, "one size does not fit all!"

Quercetin
(Chemical-Formula-C15H10O7)

Is a powerful antioxidant (available in many foods) and combats free radicals in the body. It is thought to be a powerful anti-inflammatory agent and may help to eradicate many problems associated with inflammation such as joint swelling, skin inflammation and various allergic reactions.

CHAPTER 14-BLACK PEPPERCORNS
BLACK PEPPERCORNS (Piper Nigrum)

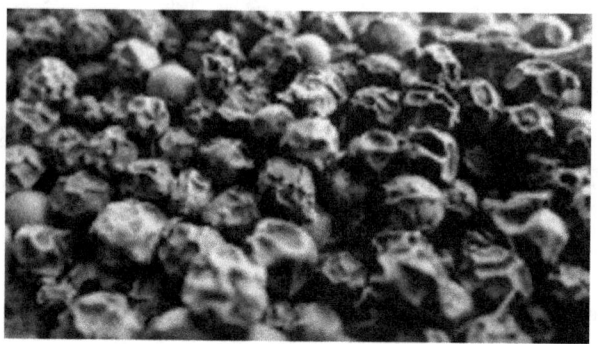

Black pepper comes from the pepper plant (Piper Nigrum) which is from the genus **Piperaceae**. It grows on a vine in the same way as grapes but it can grow very long. The vine bears little bunches of white flowers and over a long period of time in a tropical climate, they develop into berries. These are known as peppercorns. Ground peppercorns produce the spice we call pepper. Research indicates that Black Peppercorns are the most sought after spice in the world but whether this is an actual fact or not, they are highly regarded in Traditional Indian Medicine and other folk medicines as a cure for many ailments. It is also thought to help break down fat cells. It is definitely a digestive aid as the effect of pepper on the sensory parts of the mouth signal the increase of Hydrochloric Acid in the stomach which helps the digestion and faster elimination of food. Thus the digested food is processed more quickly and prevents reflux.

Another type of elimination is through the sweat glands and the heat of the pepper can cause perspiration and so clears the toxins from the skin.

Rich in dietary fibre, antioxidants and phytochemicals it boasts an array of beneficial chemicals listed below;

Manganese
(Chemical-Formula-MnO2)

is a mineral naturally occurring in our bodies in very small amounts however it is generally agreed that this amount needs to be annexed by our dietary intake. Manganese acts as a partner agent in the production of my complicated enzymes such as manganese super oxide dismutase enzyme which is another antioxidant responsible for stopping cellular damage by free radicals. It is also involved in the production of Collagen, an essential protein for healthy skin, the musculoskeletal system and the exterior protection of some organs.

Vitamin-K
(Chemical-Formula - C31H46O2)

This vitamin is actually known as vitamin K1 as there are several forms of this vitamin. Only K1 is mentioned here as it is the one which is synthesized from plants.
Vitamin K is necessary to synthesize proteins involved in blood clotting and is also essential for the synthesis of certain other proteins such as those involved in building strong bones.

Copper
(Chemical-Formula - Cu)

Copper is not produced by the body but is essential to include in our diet. In past times people used to use copper vessels to drink or cook because they knew it was needed in our diet. The practice of wearing copper on the body was common as it was believed to reduce the symptoms of Arthritis etc. Its synergy with other chemicals in the body does in fact result in reducing the symptomatic swelling and pain of Arthritis. It works in conjunction with iron to help produce a greater amount of red blood cells, thus helping to prevent anaemia and the resultant lack of energy and zest for life. Copper has an effect on the health of many organs and tissues and seems to be a factor in preventing age related symptoms

Calcium
(Chemical-Formula - Ca)

is available from many foods but processed food consumption may lessen our chances of providing the body with the amount of this essential chemical it needs to promote healthy bones and teeth. Calcium is needed for healthy growth and also to combat age related weaknesses such as Osteoporosis. Some research indicates that it may have a role in combating or preventing some types of cancer.

Chromium
(Chemical-Formula - Cr)

Chromium is only used by the body in very tiny amounts however even though this is the case it is essential in the process of metabolizing fats, carbohydrates and proteins and other biochemical processes such as the regulation of blood sugar and helps insulin perform its function.

Iron
(Chemical-Formula-Fe)

is an integral part of red blood cells, responsible for carrying oxygen to various parts of the body. Iron helps the metabolism of proteins. A deficiency of iron will necessarily result in anaemia because it lessens the production of red blood cells. For these same reasons it will obviously affect the proper function of every organ and cell in the body which rely on oxygen rich red blood cells for nourishment.

Piperine
(Chemical-Formula - C17H19NO3)

is found in Black Peppercorns and it increases the bioavailabity of Curcumin found in Turmeric, hence why I include Black Peppercorns in my list of Curry ingredients.

A major discovery is that Curcumin with the aid of Piperine can have an effect on growth hormones in the brain and is thought to be helpful in the growth of new neurons in the brain and thereby possibly prevent degenerative brain diseases and possibly increase memory capacity and recall. Time and more research will increase the knowledge of this subject but presently this looks hopeful for people with depression and Alzheimer's disease etc.

CONCLUSION

As I have chosen a list of my most often used curry vegetables and spices for discussion in this volume I am acutely aware that there are many other often used vegetables and spices that may have been discussed. I have chosen not to include these as the intention of this text is to open the reader's mind to the fact that these ingredients and many more are thought or known to have health giving properties and may help to alleviate or cure many medical problems. I personally believe that these or other regional ingredients have not ended up in curries by chance and that they were put together with the intention of helping the immune system which as I have previously mentioned is largely located in the gut.

New and extensive research is being conducted as time progresses and will always be subject to scrutiny in one form or another. That said, if you have any powers of deduction and you study the components of each ingredient, I believe it is self-evident that they are all required in varying amounts to sustain bodily health.

If you are not a curry lover, please bear in mind that there are lots of other recipes which use some or other of the ingredients. Finally please remember that it is never safe to take the word, either spoken or written, of anyone without investigating the subject yourself and make a decision on your own findings including adverse comments and contra-indications.

I hope I have offered enough information to enable this thought process however any mistakes (for which I apologise) are my own and cannot be attributed to anyone else.